TABLE OF CONTENTS

INTRODUCTION

The word "asthma" originates from the Greek meaning short of breath, meaning that any patient with breathlessness was asthmatic. The term was refined in the latter part of the 19th Century with the publication of a treatise by Henry Hyde Salter entitled "On Asthma and its Treatment". In this scholarly work Salter defined asthma as "Paroxysmal dyspnoea of a peculiar character with intervals of healthy respiration between attacks", a description that captures his concept of a disease in which the airways narrow due to contraction of their smooth muscle. His book contains remarkably accurate illustrations of the airways in asthma and bronchitis as well as the cellular appearance of asthmatic sputum some 30 years before Paul Ehrlich described aniline stains for eosinophils (eosin) and mast cells (toluidine blue). He also described black coffee as a treatment for asthmatic spasms, a drink with a high content of theobromine, a derivative of theophylline and theophylline itself. This extraordinary insight into asthma stems from Dr Salter himself suffering from asthma himself. Thus, by the late nineteenth century, physicians adopted the view that asthma was a distinct disease which had a specific set of causes, clinical consequences, and requirements for treatment.

The father of modern medicine in the Western World, Sir William Osler (one of the three founders of the John Hopkins Medical School in Baltimore, US) described asthma in his first (1892) edition of the textbook Principles and Practice of Medicine in the following terms:

1. Spasm of the bronchial muscles

2. Swelling of the bronchial mucous membrane

3. A special form of inflammation of the smaller bronchioles

4. Having many resemblances to hay fever

5. The affection running in families.

6. Often beginning in childhood and sometimes lasting into old age.

7. Bizarre and extraordinary variety of circumstances which at times induce a paroxysm:

a. Climate and atmosphere e.g. hay, dust, cat

b. Fright or violent emotion

c. Diet (overloading of the stomach) or certain foods

d. Cold infection

8. Sputum is distinctive: rounded gelatinous masses ("perles") and Curschmann spirals & octahedral crystals of Leyden

These insights came as a consequence of Osler's drive to connect clinical observation with pathology and physiology. Asthma was treated largely a disease of "bronchospasm" since bronchodilators that included theophylline, ephedrine, adrenaline and by the first half of the 20th century, isoprenaline to be followed by the selective β2-adrenoceptor agonists, salbutamol, terbutaline, remiterol and fenoterol by inhalation and as oral medications. However, their very effectiveness in reversing bronchospasm and their initial apparent safety led to their unrestricted use as over-the-counter medications. Over-reliance on bronchodilators was thought to underlie the epidemic of asthma death reported in Australia, the US and the UK that peaked in the mid-1960s (isoprenaline-related) and a second peak in New Zealand in the mid-1980s (high dose fenoterol-related).

These asthma death epidemics drew into sharp focus the shortfalls in asthma treatment and emphasised how little was understood about why the airways of asthmatics were so liable to bronchospasm. Although since the early 1920s asthma death was known to be associated with extensive inflammation and structural changes in the airways, very little was known about why this occurred and what relation it had to episodic bronchospasm. Indeed, asthma was largely managed as an acute disorder of episodic exacerbations. The discovery of reagin by Prausnitz and Küstner in 1921 as a serum substance that could passively transfer allergy to a specific agent (in this case cod allergen) subsequently led to the identification of IgE as the 5th immunoglobulin class IgE by Johansson and Ishizaka and provided the crucial link. It turned out that most asthmatics exhibited allergy to a wide range of indoor and outdoor agents including dust mites, pollens and animal proteins.

THE BIRTH OF ASTHMA AS AN INFLAMMATORY DISORDER

Thus, by the 1980s a clearer understanding of how allergen exposure triggered chemical mediator release from airway mast cells (early reaction) and this resulted in turn led to the recruitment of eosinophils, basophils and mononuclear cells (late reaction), the latter response being associated with enhanced airway reactivity to irritant stimuli (bronchial hyper responsiveness ??BHR). The allergic paradigm for asthma also explained why the mast cell stabilizing agent, sodium cromoglicate, attenuated both the allergen-induced early and late bronchoconstrictor responses. Clinical trials in the 1970s had also established that inhaled corticosteroids, notably beclomethasone dipropionate? BDP, was a highly effective controller drug for asthma when taken daily. The discovery that BDP reduced airway eosinophilic, mast cell and mononuclear cell inflammation and abrogated the late asthmatic reaction and accompanying BHR with allergen challenge created a mechanistic reason for their efficacy in controlling day-to-day asthma.

The mast cell had assumed centre stage as the principle triggering cell of asthma involving IgE-dependent activation with secretion of a wide array of autacoid, enzyme and proteoglycan mediators. However, little was known about how mast cell activation-secretion coupling occurred. Changes in Ca^{++} flux was considered important as confirmed by the inhibitory effects of Ca^{++} channel blockers such as nifedipine. You Young Kim, while on a Research Fellowship in my laboratory in 1983, showed that the lack of stimulus-related specificity and the high drug concentrations required suggested that classical calcium channel blockade was not responsible for the inhibition of mast cell mediator release observed. Although in the early 1980s histamine, prostaglandin D2, the cysteinyl leukotrienes [LTC4, LTD4 and LTE4 - previously known as slow reacting substance of anaphylaxis (SRS-A)], tryptase, chymase, heparin and exoglycosidases were all identified mast cell products with discrete proinflammatory effects, almost nothing was known about why mast cells were so sensitive to stimulation in asthma. At that time there was increasing interest in the role of T lymphocytes in underpinning the allergic response. A large number of poorly characterized factors had been traced back to lymphocytes such as neutrophil chemotactic factor, eosinophil chemotactic factor, macrophage inhibitory and activation factors, the underlying connection between these and the allergic phenotype remained a mystery.

ASTHMA

Asthma is a long-term condition affecting the airways. It involves inflammation and narrowing inside the lungs, which restricts air supply. A person with asthma may experience:

- Tightness in the chest

- Wheezing

- Breathlessness

- Coughing

- Increased mucus production

An asthma attack occurs when the symptoms become severe. Attacks can begin suddenly and range from mild to life threatening.

Most children and adults with asthma have times when their breathing becomes more difficult.

Some people with severe asthma may have breathing problems most of the time. The most common symptoms of asthma are:

- Wheezing (a whistling sound when breathing)

- Breathlessness

- A tight chest – it may feel like a band is tightening around it

- Coughing

Many things can cause these symptoms, but they're more likely to be asthma if they:

- happen often and keep coming back

- are worse at night and early in the morning

- seem to happen in response to an asthma trigger like exercise or an allergy

(such as to pollen or animal fur)

See a GP if you think you or your child may have asthma, or you have asthma and are finding it hard to control.

ASTHMA ATTACKS

Asthma can sometimes get worse for a short time – this is known as an asthma attack. It can happen suddenly, or gradually over a few days. Signs of a severe asthma attack include:

• Wheezing, coughing and chest tightness becoming severe and constant

• Being too breathless to eat, speak or sleep

• Breathing faster

• a fast heartbeat

• Drowsiness, confusion, exhaustion or dizziness

• Blue lips or fingers

• Fainting

In some cases, swelling in the airways can prevent oxygen from reaching the lungs. This means that oxygen cannot enter the bloodstream or reach vital organs. Therefore, people who experience severe symptoms need urgent medical attention. A doctor can prescribe suitable treatments and advise a person on the best ways to manage their asthma symptoms.

TYPES OF ASTHMA

Asthma can occur in many different ways and for many different reasons, but the triggers are often the same. They include airborne pollutants, viruses, pet dander, mold, and cigarette smoke.

The sections below list some common types of asthma.

CHILDHOOD ASTHMA

Asthma is the most common chronic condition in children. It can develop at any age, but it is slightly more common in children than in adults.

In 2017, children aged 5–14 years were most likely to experience asthma. In this age group, the condition affected 9.7% of people. It also affected 4.4% of children aged 0–4 years.

In the same year, asthma affected 7.7% of people aged 18 years and over.

According to the American Lung Association, some common triggers of childhood asthma include:

• Respiratory infections and colds

• Cigarette smoke, including secondhand tobacco smoke

• Allergens

• Air pollutants, including ozone and particle pollution, both indoors and outside

• Exposure to cold air

• Sudden changes in temperature

• Excitement

• Stress

• Exercise

It is vital to seek medical attention if a child starts to experience asthma, as it can be life threatening. A doctor can advise on some of the best ways to manage the condition. In some cases, asthma may improve as the child reaches adulthood. For many people, however, it is a lifelong condition.

ADULT-ONSET ASTHMA

Asthma can develop at any age, including during adulthood. According to one 2013 study, adults are more likely than children to have persistent symptoms.

Some factors that affect the risk of developing asthma in adulthood include:

- Respiratory illness

- Allergies and exposure to allergens

- Hormonal factors

- Obesity

- Stress

- Smoking

OCCUPATIONAL ASTHMA

Occupational asthma results from exposure to an allergen or irritant present in the workplace.

In the following workplaces, allergens may cause asthma in those with a sensitivity or allergy:

• Bakeries, flour mills, and kitchens

• Hospitals and other healthcare settings

• Pet shops, zoos, and laboratories where animals are present

• Farms and other agricultural settings

In the following occupations, irritants can trigger asthma symptoms:

• Car repairs and manufacturing

• Engineering and metalwork

• Woodwork and carpentry

• Electronics and assembly industries

• Hairdressing salons

• Indoor swimming pools

Those with a higher risk include people who:

• Smoke

• have allergic rhinitis

• Have a history of asthma or environmental allergies

A person's work environment can trigger a return of childhood asthma or the start of adult-onset asthma.

DIFFICULT-TO-CONTROL AND SEVERE ASTHMA

Research suggests that around 5–10% of people with asthma have severe asthma.

Some people have severe symptoms for reasons that do not relate directly to asthma. For example, they may not yet have learned the correct way to use an inhaler.

Others have severe refractory asthma. In these cases, the asthma does not respond to treatment — even with high dosages of medication or the correct use of inhalers. This type of asthma may affect 3.6% of people with the condition, according to one 2015 study.

Eosinophilic asthma is another type of asthma that, in severe cases, may not respond to the usual medications. Although some people with eosinophilic asthma manage with standard asthma medications, others may benefit from specific "biologic" therapies. One type of biologic medication reduces the numbers of eosinophils, which are a type of blood cell involved in an allergic reaction that can trigger asthma.

SEASONAL ASTHMA

This type of asthma occurs in response to allergens that are only in the surrounding environment at certain times of year. For example, cold air in the winter or pollen in the spring or summer may trigger symptoms of seasonal asthma.

People with seasonal asthma still have the condition for the rest of the year, but they usually do not experience symptoms. Asthma does not always stem from an allergy, however.

CAUSES AND TRIGGERS

Health professionals do not know exactly what causes asthma, but genetic and environmental factors both seem to play significant roles. Some factors, such as sensitization to an allergen, may be both causes and triggers. The sections below list some others.

Pregnancy

According to one study, smoking during pregnancy appears to increase the risk of the fetus developing asthma later in life. Some women also experience an aggravation of asthma symptoms while pregnant.

Obesity

One article from 2014 suggested that there seem to be higher levels of asthma in people with obesity than those without it. The authors note that, in one study, children with obesity who lost weight also saw improvements in their asthma symptoms.

There is now a growing body of evidence suggesting that both conditions involve a chronic inflammatory response, and this could explain the link.

Allergies

Allergies develop when a person's body becomes sensitized to a specific substance. Once the sensitization has taken place, the person will be susceptible to an allergic reaction each time they come into contact with the substance. Not every person with asthma has an allergy, but there is often a link. In people with allergic disease, exposure to specific allergens can trigger symptoms. One 2013 study found that 60–80% of children and young adults with asthma are sensitive to at least one allergen.

Smoking tobacco

Cigarette smoking can trigger asthma symptoms, according to the American Lung Association.

Asthma, even without smoking, can cause damage to the lungs. This can increase the risk of developing various tobacco-related lung conditions, such as chronic obstructive pulmonary disease, and it can make symptoms more severe.

Environmental factors

Air pollution, both inside the home and outside of it, can affect the development and triggers of asthma. Some allergens inside the home include:

• Mold

• Dust

• Animal hair and dander

• fumes from household cleaners and paints

• Cockroaches

• Feathers

Other triggers in the home and outdoors include:

• Pollen

• Air pollution from traffic and other sources

• Ground-level ozone

Stress

Stress can give rise to asthma symptoms, but so can several other emotions. Joy, anger, excitement, laughter, crying, and other emotional reactions can all trigger an asthma attack. Scientists have also found evidence to suggest that asthma may be more likely in people with mental health conditions such as depression. Others have suggested that long-term stress may lead to epigenetic changes that result in chronic asthma.

Genetic factors

There is evidence to suggest that asthma runs in families. Recently, scientists have mapped out some of the genetic changes that may play a role in its development.

In some cases, epigenetic changes are responsible. These occur when an environmental factor causes a gene to change.

Hormonal factors

Around 5.5% of males and 9.7% of females have asthma. In addition, symptoms may vary according to a female's reproductive stage and point in the menstrual cycle.

For example, during their reproductive years, symptoms may worsen during menstruation, compared with other times of the month. Doctors call this perimenstrual asthma. During menopause, however, asthma symptoms may improve.

Some scientists believe that hormonal activity may impact immune activity, resulting in hypersensitivity in the airways. People with intermittent asthma may also have symptoms only some of the time

ASTHMA TREATMENTS

There's currently no cure for asthma, but treatment can help control the symptoms so you're able to live a normal, active life.

Inhalers – devices that let you breathe in medicine – are the main treatment. Tablets and other treatments may also be needed if your asthma is severe. You'll usually create a personal action plan with a doctor or asthma nurse. This includes information about your medicines, how to monitor your condition and what to do if you have an asthma attack.

Inhalers

Inhalers can help:

• Relieve symptoms when they occur (reliever inhalers)

• Stop symptoms developing (preventer inhalers)

Some people need an inhaler that does both (combination inhalers).

Reliever inhalers

Most people with asthma will be given a reliever inhaler. These are usually blue. You use a reliever inhaler to treat your symptoms when they occur. They should relieve your symptoms within a few minutes.

Tell a GP or asthma nurse if you have to use your reliever inhaler 3 or more times a week. They may suggest additional treatment, such as a preventer inhaler. Reliever inhalers have few side effects, but they can sometimes cause shaking or a fast heartbeat for a few minutes after they're used.

Preventer inhalers

If you need to use a reliever inhaler often, you may also need a preventer inhaler.

You use a preventer inhaler every day to reduce the inflammation and sensitivity of your airways, which stops your symptoms occurring. It's important to use it even when you do not have symptoms. Speak to a GP or asthma nurse if you continue to have symptoms while using a preventer inhaler.

Preventer inhalers contain steroid medicine.

They do not usually have side effects, but can sometimes cause:

• A fungal infection of the mouth or throat (oral thrush)

• A hoarse voice

• A sore throat

You can help prevent these side effects by using a spacer, which is a hollow plastic tube you attach to your inhaler, as well as by rinsing your mouth or cleaning your teeth after using your inhaler.

Combination inhalers

If using reliever and preventer inhalers does not control your asthma, you may need an inhaler that combines both. Combination inhalers are used every day to help stop symptoms occurring and provide long-lasting relief if they do occur.

It's important to use it regularly, even if you do not have symptoms. Side effects of combination inhalers are similar to those of reliever and preventer inhalers.

Tablets

You may also need to take tablets if using an inhaler alone is not helping control your symptoms.

Leukotriene receptor antagonists (LTRAs)

LTRAs are the main tablets used for asthma. They also come in syrup and powder form. You take them every day to help stop your symptoms occurring. Possible side effects include tummy aches and headaches.

Theophylline

Theophylline may also be recommended if other treatments are not helping to control your symptoms. It's taken every day to stop your symptoms occurring. Possible side effects include headaches and feeling sick.

Steroid tablets

Steroid tablets may be recommended if other treatments are not helping to control your symptoms. They can be taken either:

• As an immediate treatment when you have an asthma attack

• Every day as a long-term treatment to prevent symptoms – this is usually only necessary if you have very severe asthma and inhalers do not control your symptoms

Long-term or frequent use of steroid tablets can occasionally cause side effects such as:

• Increased appetite, leading to weight gain

• Easy bruising

• Mood changes

• Fragile bones (osteoporosis)

• High blood pressure

You'll be monitored regularly while taking steroid tablets to check for signs of any problems.

OTHER TREATMENTS

Other treatments, such as injections or surgery, are rarely needed, but may be recommended if all other treatments are not helping.

Injections

For some people with severe asthma, injections given every few weeks can help control the symptoms. The main injections for asthma are:

• Benralizumab (Fasenra)

• Omalizumab (Xolair)

• Mepolizumab (Nucala)

• Reslizumab (Cinqaero)

These medicines are not suitable for everyone with asthma and can only be prescribed by an asthma specialist. The main side effect is discomfort where the injection is given.

Surgery

A procedure called bronchial thermoplasty may be offered as a treatment for severe asthma. It works well and there are no serious concerns about its safety.

You will be sedated or put to sleep using a general anesthetics during a bronchial thermoplasty. It involves passing a thin, flexible tube down your throat and into your lungs. Heat is then used on the muscles around the airways to help stop them narrowing and causing asthma symptoms.

Complementary therapies

Several complementary therapies have been suggested as possible treatments for asthma, including:

• Breathing exercises – such as techniques called the Papworth method and the Buteyko method

- Traditional Chinese herbal medicine

- Acupuncture

- Ionisers – devices that use an electric current to charge molecules of air

- Manual therapies – such as chiropractic

- Homeopathy

- Dietary supplements

There's little evidence to suggest many of these treatments help.

There's some evidence that breathing exercises can improve symptoms and reduce the need for reliever medicines in some people, but they should not be used instead of your medicine.

Work-related asthma

If you seem to have occupational asthma, where your asthma is linked to your job, you'll be referred to a specialist to confirm the diagnosis.

If your employer has an occupational health service, they should also be informed, along with your health and safety officer.

Your employer has a responsibility to protect you from the causes of occupational asthma. It may sometimes be possible to:

- substitute or remove the substance that's triggering your asthma from your workplace

- Redeploy you to another role within the company

- Provide you with protective breathing equipment

DIET

Does the word "diet" immediately make you think of an unpleasant weight-loss regimen? If it did, you are probably not alone.For example, consider the use of the term "diet" in marketing food products it usually describes foods low in calories, such as diet soda. But there is another meaning of this word.Diet can also refer to the food and drink a person consumes daily and the mental and physical circumstances connected to eating. Nutrition involves more than simply eating a "good" diet it is about nourishment on every level.It involves relationships with family, friends, nature (the environment), our bodies, our community, and the world.

BALANCE DIET

A balanced diet is one that fulfills all of a person's nutritional needs.Humans need a certain amount of calories and nutrients to stay healthy.A balanced diet provides all the nutrients a person requires, without going over the recommended daily calorie intake.By eating a balanced diet, people can get the nutrients and calories they need and avoid eating junk food, or food without nutritional value.

The United States Department of Agriculture (USDA) used to recommend following a food pyramid. However, as nutritional science has changed, they now recommend eating foods from the five groups and building a balanced plate.According to the USDA's recommendations, half of a person's plate should consist of fruits and vegetables.The other half should be made up of grains and protein.They recommend accompanying each meal with a serving of low-fat dairy or another source of the nutrients found in dairy.

THE 5 FOOD GROUPS

A healthful, balanced diet includes foods from these five groups:

• Vegetables

• Fruits

• Grains

• Protein

• Dairy

Vegetables

The vegetable group includes five subgroups:

• Leafy greens

• Red or orange vegetables

• Starchy vegetables

• Beans and peas (legumes)

• Other vegetables, such as eggplant or zucchini

To get enough nutrients and keep dietary boredom at bay, people should choose a variety of vegetables. Additionally, the USDA recommend that people eat vegetables from each of the five subgroups every week.

People may enjoy vegetables raw or cooked. However, it is important to remember that cooking vegetables removes some of their nutritional value. Also, some methods, such as deep-frying, can add unhealthful fats to a dish.

Fruits

A balanced diet also includes plenty of fruit.Instead of getting fruit from juice, nutrition expert's recommend eating whole fruits.

Juice contains fewer nutrients. Also, the manufacturing process often adds empty calories due to added sugar. People should opt for fresh or frozen fruits, or fruits canned in water instead of syrup.

Grains

There are two subgroups: whole grains and refined grains.

Whole grains include all three parts of the grain, which are the bran, germ, and endosperm.The body breaks down whole grains slowly, so they have less effect on a person's blood sugar. Additionally, whole grains tend to contain more fiber and protein than refined grains.

Refined grains are processed and do not contain the three original components. Refined grains also tend to have less protein and fiber, and they can cause blood sugar spikes.

Grains used to form the base of the government-approved food pyramid, meaning that most of a person's daily caloric intake came from grains. However, the updated guidelines suggest that grains should make up only a quarter of a person's plate.

At least half of the grains that a person eats daily should be whole grains.Healthful whole grains include:

• Quinoa

• Oats

• Brown rice

• Barley

• Buckwheat

Protein

The 2015–2020 Dietary Guidelines for Americans state that all people should include nutrient-dense protein as part of their regular diet.The guidelines suggest that this protein should make up a quarter of a person's plate.

Nutritious protein choices include:

• Lean beef and pork

• Chicken and turkey

• Fish

• Beans, peas, and legumes

Dairy

Dairy and fortified soy products are a vital source of calcium.The USDA recommend consuming low-fat versions whenever possible.

Low-fat dairy and soy products include:

• Ricotta or cottage cheese

• Low-fat milk

• Yogurt

• Soy milk

People who are lactose intolerant can opt for low-lactose or lactose-free products, or choose soy-based sources of calcium and other nutrients.

Losing Weight

A poor diet is a common reason why people struggle with weight loss.When combined with a regular exercise routine, a balanced diet can help a person reduce their risk factors for obesity or gaining weight.

A balanced diet can help a person lose weight by:

• Increasing their protein intake

• Avoiding excessive carbohydrates or processed foods

• Getting essential nutrients, including minerals, vitamins, and fiber

• Preventing binge eating

For some people, adding 30 minutes of walking each day and making minor changes, such as taking the stairs, can help them burn calories and lose weight.

For those that can, adding moderate exercise that includes cardio and resistance training will help speed weight loss.

DIETS THAT ARE SUPPORTED BY SCIENCE

While many diets may work for you, the key is finding one you like and can stick to in the long run.

1. Low-Carb, Whole-Food Diet

The low-carb, whole-food diet is perfect for people who need to lose weight, optimize health, and lower their risk of disease.It's flexible, allowing you to fine-tune your carb intake depending on your goals. This diet is high in vegetables, meat, fish, eggs, fruits, nuts, and fats but low in starches, sugars, and processed foods.

2. Mediterranean diet

The Mediterranean diet is an excellent diet that has been thoroughly studied.It's particularly effective for heart disease prevention. It emphasizes foods that were commonly eaten around the Mediterranean region during the 20th century and earlier. As such, it includes plenty of vegetables, fruits, fish, poultry, whole grains, legumes, dairy products, and extra virgin olive oil.

HOW TO DIET

Low carb, the 5:2 diet, detox, cabbage soup... there's no shortage of novelty diet programmes promising to help you lose weight fast. The big question is, do they work?Most do lead to fast – sometimes dramatic – weight loss, but only for the pounds to creep back on again at the end of the diet.

More worryingly, many fad diets are based on dodgy science or no research at all, prescribing eating practices that are unhealthy and can make you ill.

The British Dietetic Association says there's no "wonder-diet you can follow without some associated nutritional or health risk".

A fad diet is typically a low calorie diet with few foods or an unusual combination of foods.People can lose weight very quickly initially, but soon get fed up and return to old eating habits, and end up putting the weight back on.

Reasons To Avoid Fad Diets

1. Some Diets Can Make You Ill

Many diets, especially crash diets, are geared to dramatically reducing the number of calories you consume. Crash diets make you feel very unwell and unable to function properly, because they're nutritionally unbalanced, crash diets can lead to long-term poor health.

2. Excluding Foods Is Dangerous

Some diets recommend cutting out certain foods, such as meat, and fish, wheat or dairy products. Cutting out certain food groups altogether could prevent you getting the important nutrients and vitamins your body needs to function properly. You can lose weight without cutting out foods from your diet.

3. Low-Carb Diets Can Be High In Fat

Some diets are very low in carbohydrates (like pasta, bread and rice), which are an important source of energy. While you may lose weight on these types of diets, they're often high in protein and fat, which can make you ill.

Low-carbohydrate diets can also cause side effects such as bad breath, headaches and constipation.

It's been suggested that the high protein content of these diets 'dampens' the appetite and feelings of hunger. Many low-carbohydrate diets allow you to eat foods high in saturated fat, such as butter, cheese and meat. Too much saturated fat can raise your cholesterol and increase your risk of heart disease and stroke.

4. Detox Diets Don't Work

Detox diets are based on the idea that toxins build up in the body and can be removed by eating, or not eating, certain things. But there's no evidence that toxins build up in our bodies.If they did, we'd feel very ill.

Detox diets may lead to weight loss because they involve restricting calories, cutting out certain foods altogether, such as wheat or dairy, and eating a very limited range of foods.

5. Cabbage Soup, Blood Group, The 5:2 Diet And Other Fad Diets Are Often Far-Fetched

Some fad diets are based on eating a single food or meal, such as cabbage soup, chocolate or eggs. Others recommend eating foods only in particular combinations based on your genetic type or blood group. Often there's little or no evidence to back up these diets, and they can be difficult to keep to in the long term.

If followed over long periods, these diets can be very unbalanced and bad for your health. You may lose weight in the short term, but it's much better to lose weight gradually and to be healthy.

HOW TO LOSE WEIGHT THE HEALTHY WAY

We put on weight when the amount of calories we eat exceeds the amount of calories we burn through normal everyday activities and exercise.Most adults need to eat less and get more active. The only way to lose weight healthily and keep it off is to make permanent changes to the way you eat and exercise.

A few small alterations, such as eating less and choosing drinks that are lower in fat, sugar and alcohol, can help you lose weight.There are also plenty of ways to make physical activity part of your life.If you're overweight, aim to lose about 5 to 10% of your starting weight by losing 0.5 to 1kg (1 to 2lb) a week.

You should be able to lose this amount if you eat about 500 to 600 fewer calories than you normally consume each day. An average man needs about 2,500 calories a day and an average woman about 2,000 calories to stay the same weight.

DIET AND ASTHMA

It's no secret that a well-balanced diet keeps the body and mind strong and healthy. Eating the right foods and nutrients can give us energy to stay active throughout the day, supports our immune system and improve our health—even our lung health!

The right nutrients in your diet can help you breathe easier, and in some cases, help minimize asthma symptoms. While there's no specific diet recommendation for asthma, there are some foods and nutrients that may help support lung function and reduce asthma symptoms.

HOW DOES FOOD RELATE TO BREATHING?

Metabolism is the process of changing food to fuel in the body. Oxygen is important in this process to help burn the food's nutrient molecules. When sugars, fibers, fats and proteins are broken down, energy is the final product. Carbon dioxide is created as a waste product and is exhaled.

Different types of nutrients require different amounts of oxygen and produce different amounts of carbon dioxide. Carbohydrates use more oxygen and produce more carbon dioxide, whereas fats produce less carbon dioxide for the amount of oxygen consumed. "Some people with COPD feel that eating a diet with fewer carbohydrates and more healthy fats helps them breathe easier," says Traci Gonzales, nurse practitioner and volunteer spokesperson for the American Lung Association.

WHAT CAN HELP

Vitamin D: Vitamin D plays an important role in boosting immune system responses and helps to reduce airway inflammation. Low levels of vitamin D have been linked to increased risk of asthma attacks in children and adults. Research also shows adults with asthma may benefit from vitamin D supplements, such as protective effects against acute respiratory infection and reduced rate of exacerbations needing treatment with systemic corticosteroids.

Food sources of vitamin D include: fortified milk, salmon, orange juice and eggs.

Vitamin E: Vitamin E contains a chemical compound called tocopherol, which may decrease the risk of some asthma symptoms like coughing or wheezing.

Sources of vitamin E include: almonds, raw seeds, Swiss chard, mustard greens, kale, broccoli and hazelnuts.

WHAT TO AVOID

Sulfites: While some fresh fruit such as apples or bananas can be helpful in your diet, sulfites are found in many dried fruits and can cause an adverse reaction or even worsen asthma symptoms for some.

Sulfites are also found in some pickled food, shrimp, maraschino cherries, bottled lemon or lime juices and alcohol. "Not everyone knows about this connection," says Gonzales. "I've seen quite a few people whose asthma can be triggered when drinking alcohol, particularly red wine."

Foods that cause gas: Avoid foods that cause gas or bloating, which often make breathing more difficult. This may cause chest tightness and trigger asthma flare ups.

Foods to avoid include: beans, carbonated drinks, onions, garlic and fried foods.

Salicylates: Salicylates are naturally occurring chemical compounds and, although it's rare, some people with asthma may be sensitive to salicylates found in tea, coffee, some herbs or spices and even aspirin, according to Gonzales.

People with common food allergies or sensitivities, such as dairy products, artificial ingredients, tree nuts, wheat or shellfish, may also be at risk of developing asthma.

Some asthma patients may have heard of soy isoflavone supplements as a possible remedy for symptoms. A study from the American Lung Association Airways Clinical Research Centers (ACRC) Network has found that use of a soy isoflavone supplement did not result in improved lung function or clinical outcomes, including symptoms, episodes of poor asthma control or airway inflammation.

Keep in mind that food restrictions and allergies vary depending on the individual. Remember, no single food or vitamin will supply all the nutrients you need. A diet with a variety of vitamins and nutrients that keep our minds and bodies healthy.

It's important to consult your doctor or a nutritionist before making any drastic changes to your diet.

Foods rarely trigger an asthma attack. But the symptoms of a severe allergic reaction to some foods can mimic asthma symptoms. The first step is to know if you have a food allergy. Any abnormal reaction to a food is considered an adverse reaction. Adverse reactions can either be:

• Food allergy: When your immune system reacts to proteins in foods that usually are safe or harmless. Your doctor can do skin tests to find out if you're sensitive to certain foods.

• Food intolerance: When your body responds to the food, not your immune system. Examples include food poisoning, reactions to chemicals in food or drinks such as caffeine, or reflux.

The most common foods associated with allergic symptoms are:

• Eggs

• Cow's milk

• Peanuts

• Soy

• Wheat

• Fish

• Shrimp and other shellfish

• Tree nuts

FOOD PRESERVATIVES AND ASTHMA

Food preservatives can also trigger an asthma attack. Additives, such as sodium bisulfite, potassium bisulfite, sodium metabisulfite, potassium metabisulfite, and sodium sulfite, are commonly used in food processing or preparation and can be found in foods such as:

- Dried fruits or vegetables

- Potatoes (packaged and some prepared)

- Wine and beer

- Bottled lime or lemon juice

- Shrimp (fresh, frozen, or prepared)

- Pickled foods

SYMPTOMS OF FOOD ALLERGIES AND ASTHMA

For most people, the usual symptoms of food allergies are hives, rash, nausea, vomiting, and diarrhea. If you have food allergies that trigger symptoms of an asthma attack, you will likely have these allergy symptoms, followed by coughing and wheezing. And if not caught quickly, anaphylaxis -- swelling of the throat, cutting off your airway -- may result.

If you suspect certain foods are asthma triggers for you, talk to your doctor. They can give you allergy skin tests to find out if you're allergic to these foods.

WHAT SHOULD I DO IF I HAVE FOOD ALLERGIES AND ASTHMA?

There are simple ways to say safe:

• Avoid the food trigger. Try not to come into contact with the food you're allergic to. Always read labels and ask how foods are prepared when you eat out.

• Consider allergy shots. They can train your immune system to not overreact. The doctors will give you allergy shots (immunotherapy) -- a small amount of the substance that causes your allergy. After repeated shots over a period of time, your immune system eventually stops causing the allergic reaction. Ask your doctor if you're a candidate for allergy shots. Sublingual immunotherapy (SLIT) is an alternative to allergy shots. You let the medicine dissolve under your tongue instead of getting a shot.

• Keep epinephrine with you. If your allergies are severe, you should keep two epinephrine shot kits with you that are always easy to get to. If you have any sign of anaphylaxis, don't hesitate to use the epinephrine auto-injector, even if you aren't sure your symptoms are allergy-related. Using the auto-injector as a precaution won't hurt you and might save you. Dial 911 after you give yourself the shot.

DIET GUIDELINES

Do not overeat

Only eat when you feel hungry. Eating when you are not hungry means that your body uses energy in order to process food that it does not need. This leads to increased breathing and is not good for your health. Do not eat just because it is a particular time of the day. It is very important to adhere to this in order to help increase your control pause.

Stop eating when you feel you have had enough. Overeating will increase the risk factors for chronic degenerative disease such as cancer, diabetes, heart disease, and arthritic diseases. It has been well documented that reducing food intake will promote longevity of life. Reducing calorie intake while meeting your body's requirements of nutrients is the secret to a better and longer life. 'More die in the United States of too much food than too little'.

Do not eat for a couple of hours before going to bed. If you have something to eat or a protein drink before you go to bed this will cause deep breathing during the night, will result in poor sleep and possible waking from symptoms. Sumo wrestlers intentionally have a large meal before they sleep in order to accumulate weight. The exact same process is happening to us, albeitunintentionally.

Reduce your protein intake

It should be a priority to reduce or eliminate dairy produce entirely from your diet because it can be mucus producing and may contribute to many allergies and breathing problems. Children with nasal congestion and runny noses often experience a great improvement when they stop drinking cow'smilk. While this will not apply to all people in general, it does seem to apply to many people with asthma. Asian countries have very low dairy consumption due to lactose intolerance and their asthma rate is non existent compared with ours.

If a person is lactose intolerant, dairy products are not a good source of calcium because the body is unable to absorb the calcium from milk sources.

If dairy is such a good provider, then why is osteoporosis often higher in countries with the highest dairy consumption? Cow's milk is specially formulated and should be used only as nature intended which is to feed and develop calves. Milk is not the only food source to provide calcium. Good sources of calcium include kelp, turnip greens, rhubarb, broccoli, lambs kidney, tofu, tinned salmon with bones, baked beans, fortified oatmeal and other cereals, and all leafy green vegetables. Turnip greens provide an estimated twice as much calcium as milk. A question often asked is this: what is there left to eat for breakfast if milk is eliminated from the diet? Your morning meal is to break your fast from the day before and to start your new day. Advertising and marketing gurus have unfortunately re-educated the masses to eat stale processed sugary foods for this important meal. Always remember that the foods which are widely advertised are usually processed foods. The best meal by far, which fed our ancestors for generations, is porridge. It provides essential fibre, energy and contains no additives, colouring or preservatives. Porridge cooked in the morning in water with a little honey is a good start to any day. If you are considering reducing your dairy intake, ensure that you eat green vegetables and consider calcium supplements, especially if you are taking steroids.

Limit consumption of processed foods and stimulants

Consumption of processed foods should be limited. In the 1930s Dr Weston Price conducted an interesting study of traditional groups and their change to a more processed westernised diet. 7 When the Gaelic people, living on the Hebrides off the coast of Scotland, changed from their traditional diet of small sea foods and oatmeal to the modernised diet of 'angel food cake, white bread and many white flour commodities, marmalade, canned vegetables, sweetened fruit juices, jams, and confections', first generation children became mouth breathers and their immunity from diseases of civilisation reduced dramatically.

The traditional diets were found to provide at least four times the minimum requirement of nutrients, while modern diets did not meet the minimum requirement.

Sugar affects your adrenals which produce your body's natural source of steroid. Of sugary foods, chocolate has the most harmful effect for any person with asthma. Sometimes it may not be until the following day that symptoms are experienced from the consumption of chocolate. Sugar raises blood sugar levels and causes a depletion of essential minerals such as magnesium. Interestingly, 'desserts' spelled backwards is 'stressed'.

Little is known about the real nutritional content of white bread. White flour contains little nutrition and increases mucus production. To quote Dr Price's book Nutrition and Physical Degeneration: 'Modern white flour has had approximately four fifths of the phosphorous and nearly all of the vitamins removed by processing, in order to produce a flour that can be shipped without becoming infested with insect life. Tests showed that white bread was unable to sustain insect life, while half a slice of whole rye bread was totally consumed by bugs.' This begs the significant question: how come white bread is not good enough for bugs to eat, yet is good enough for humans to eat?

Black tea and especially coffee are regarded as stimulants. The group of asthma drugs known as Xantines are based on the same properties as coffee. These drugs are not now commonly used due to their many side effects. Coffee

Eat more fresh food

Fresh food is best. Canned food is not recommended due to the contamination of the food by aluminium packaging. Frozen vegetables, while not ideal, are a better source of prepared vegetables than canned. Best of all is fresh fruit and vegetables grown without the use of pesticides or chemical fertilisers.

It is beneficial to eat five portions of fresh vegetables and fruit per day, especially greens such as cabbage, broccoli, kale and kelp because these provide good sources of magnesium and calcium. Furthermore, vegetables do not promote the formation of mucus. Lightly cooking food and vegetables provides a richer source of nutrients and has less effect on breathing. However, the more raw the food, the less the effect it has on our breathing.

Ingredients such as garlic, ginger, curry, onions and sea salt are beneficial for asthma. Garlic, ginger and onions boost the immune system, thin mucus and are very helpful for people with respiratory complaints. It is recommended that you drink a small amount of sea salt in warm water any time you have asthma symptoms and especially during the cleansing reaction.

Fruits which may not be helpful for people with asthma include oranges, grapefruits, lemons and limes as they are antigenic, i.e. they trigger an immune response. Drinking large amounts of orange juice each day may exacerbate symptoms. Bananas are mucus producing because they contain high potassium, and strawberries and raspberries increase histamine levels.

Food intolerances

There are many foods to which you can be intolerant but usually eat every day.

You may not notice the negative effect because there is a delayed reaction and symptoms run from one day into the next. Regular amounts of the offending food will ameliorate the effect of the initial consumption, resembling the alcoholic who consumes further quantities to obtain relief from his addiction.

The following foods commonly trigger symptoms: milk, eggs, peanuts, soy, wheat, fish and shellfish. Along with these are many additives such as sulphites, Tartrazine, and monosodium glutamate.

Some foods can give you direct feedback on whether they are helping you or hurting you. For example, if your nose is totally clogged after drinking a cup of coffee – then coffee does not suit you. (It is debatable whether it suits anyone.)

Testing for food intolerance does require some detective work. Some indicators of food intolerance are foods that your parents are allergic to, foods you crave and foods you eat between meals. Crisps and chocolate are the mostcommon items to fall into this category.

A good method of determining which foods you may be intolerant to is by eliminating them for a period of weeks. It is worth noting that if you cannot do without a food for twenty-one days, then you are very likely to be addicted to that food. For example, if you feel that milk exacerbates your symptoms, then for two weeks do not drink milk or consume any product which contains milk.

By then you should have noticed an improvement in your condition if milk does not agree with you. If you do decide to reintroduce an offending food into your diet, be very careful because the reaction may be far greater following a period of withdrawal. It is advisable to speak with a nutritional expert before embarking on an elimination diet.

Other tests include missing your evening meal. On waking consume a small quantity of the suspect food. If your pulse rises more than ten beats fifteen minutes after eating, then consider eliminating this food from your diet and observe if there is an improvement in your condition.